25 HEALTHY VEGAN SNACKS

COOKBOOK

LOW FAT

DIARY FREE RECIPES

QUICK AND EASY VEGAN SNACK

RECIPE

CATHERINE R. DIALS.

© 2023 by Catherine R. Dials

This book is a work of nonfiction. Any similarity to real persons, living or dead is coincidental and not intended by the author.

Table of content

INTRODUCTION

Ashley, a passionate vegan, was on a quest to create the ultimate healthy vegan snacks cookbook. She wanted to share her culinary creativity with the world and inspire others to embrace a plant-based lifestyle. With a notebook full of recipes and a heart full of enthusiasm, she embarked on her culinary journey.

From crispy kale chips to creamy avocado hummus, Ashley's kitchen became a hub of experimentation. Her friends and family eagerly volunteered to taste-test each delectable creation.

As the days turned into weeks, Ashley's cookbook took shape, and she named it "25 healthy vegan snacks cookbook. " Packed with vibrant photos and mouthwatering recipes, the book aimed to prove that vegan snacks could be both delicious and nutritious.

25 HEALTHY VEGAN SNACKS

These quick and easy vegan snack recipes are simple to do and can be adjusted with your favorite flavors and ingredients.

GUACAMOLE AND SALSA WITH HOME MADE TORTILLA CHIPS

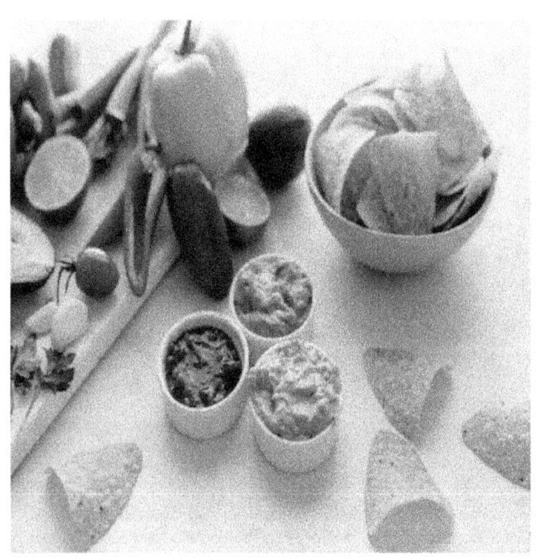

Ingredients for Guacamole

2 ripe avocados, 1 small onion, finely chopped, 2 tomatoes, dice, 1-2 cloves garlic, mince, 1 lime, juice, Salt and pepper to taste, Fresh cilantro, chopped (optional)

Ingredient for Salsa

Diced tomatoes 4-6, 1 small onion, finely chopped, 1 jalapeño pepper, seeded and finely chopped, 2 cloves garlic, minced,1 lime, juiced, Salt and pepper to taste, Fresh cilantro, chopped (optional).

Ingredients for Home made Tortilla Chips

Tortillas small corn, vegetable oil, and salt to taste.

Preparation for Guacamole

After halves the avocados, scoop the flesh into a basin.

With a fork, mash the avocados until they are smooth.

Add the minced garlic, chopped onion, diced tomatoes, lime juice, salt, pepper, and cilantro.

Combine everything, taste it, and make any necessary seasoning adjustments.

Serve with tortilla chips or fresh vegetables.

Preparation for Salsa

Mix diced tomatoes, chopped onions, minced garlic, cilantro,

Lime juice, salt, and pepper in a bowl.

Mix carefully to thoroughly combine all the ingredients.

Taste and modify the seasonings as necessary.

With tortilla chips, serve.

Preparation for Home made Tortilla Chips

The oven should be heated to 350°F (175°C).

Cut the corn tortillas into desired chip shapes before stacking them.

Place the tortilla pieces in a single layer on the baking sheet.

Spray them with cooking spray sparingly or lightly brush them

with vegetable oil.

Add salt to the tortilla chips.

Bake them until they are golden brown and crispy.

Take them out of the oven and let them cool before serving.

PEANUT BUTTER AND BANANA SANDWICH BITES

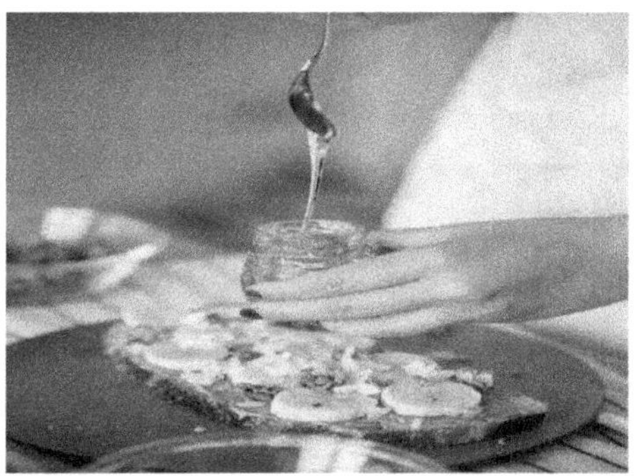

Ingredients for banana sandwich

Whole wheat bread or bread of choice, Vegan Peanut butter

and Banana, sliced into rounds.

Preparation for banana sandwich

Spread two layers of pecan butter on each of the two slices of

whole wheat bread.

Place one slice with banana rounds on it.

Make a sandwich by placing the other slice of peanut butter-covered bread on top.

Cut the sandwich into bite-sized pieces or create creative shapes with a cookware cutter and Enjoy

ROASTED CHICKPEAS WITH VARIOUS FLAVORINGS

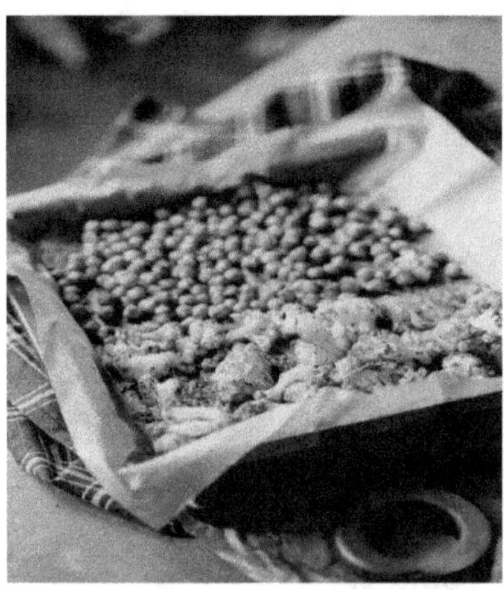

Ingredients for roasted chiken peas

1 can (15 oz) chickpeas (garbanzo beans), drained and rinsed.

1-2 tablespoons olive oil, seasonings of choice

(Paprika, cumin, Chili powder, garlic powder, salt, pepper).

Preparation for roasted chicken peas

The oven should be heated to 400°F (200°C).

Use a paper towel to gently pat the chickpeas dry to remove any excess moisture.

Toss the chickpeas in a bowl with the olive oil and your preferred seasonings.

Spread the seasoning-seasoned chickpeas in a single layer on a baking sheet.

Shake the pan occasionally as they roast in the oven for 20 to 30 minutes, or until they are crispy and golden brown.

Take out of the oven, allow it cool, and then enjoy as a crunchy snack.

FRUIT KABOBS WITH A SWEET DIPPING SAUCE

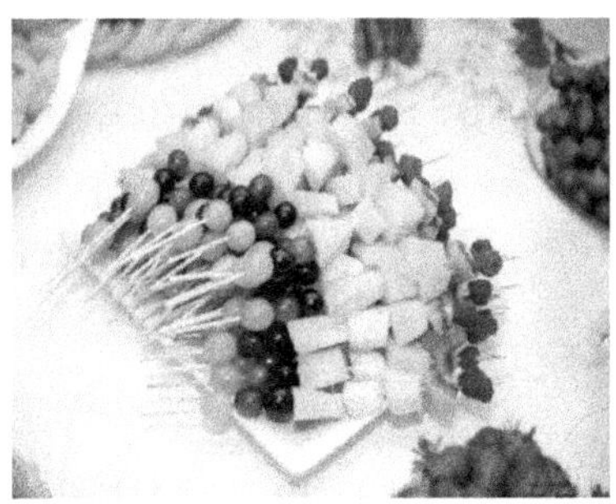

Ingredients for fruit kabob

Assorted fruits (straw berries, pineapple chunks, grapes, Melon balls), wooden skewers (soaked in water to prevent burning).

Ingredients for the Sweet Dipping Sauce

1/2 cup vegan yogurt (almond, soy, coconut), 2 tablespoons maple syrup or agave nectar, 1/2 teaspoon vanilla extract (optional).

Preparation for fruit kabob

Thread the assorted fruits onto the wooden skewers to create fruit kabobs.

Preparation for dipping sauce

For the dipping sauce, mix vegan yogurt, maple syrup, and vanilla extract in a bowl.

Serve the fruit kabobs with the sweet dipping sauce for a refreshing and healthy snack.

POPCORN

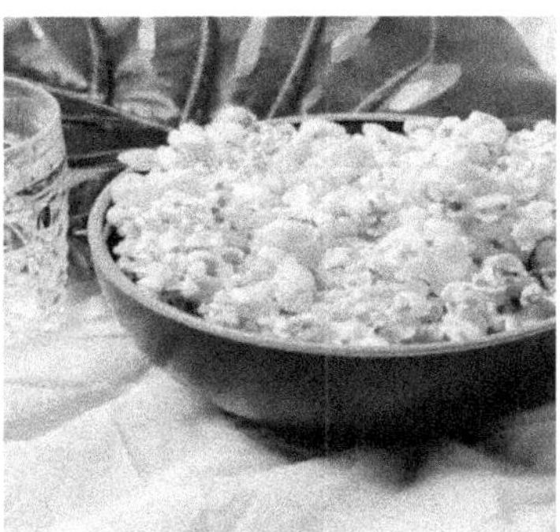

Ingredients for popcorn

Popcorn kernels, Vegetable oil, Savory seasonings (nutritional yeast, garlic powder, onion powder, smoked paprika, chili powder, salt).

Preparation for popcorn

A large saucepan with a lid should be heated over medium heat.

Add some popcorn kernels and enough vegetable oil to cover the bottom of the pot.

Place a lid on the saucepan and wait for the test kernels to pop.

This shows that the oil is sufficiently heated.

Remove the test kernels add the remaining popcorn kernels, and cover the pot.

Shake the pot often to ensure even popping and prevent burning.

Remove the pot from the heat when the popping has greatly decreased.

Mix the delicious seasonings of your choice in a separate bowl.

Sprinkle little more oil over the previously popped popcorn and toss it to evenly distribute it.

Sprinkle the seasoning mixture over the popcorn and give it another quick toss to coat.

Serve your seasoned popcorn right away for a delicious and

filling snack.

KALE CHIPS WITH NUTRITIONAL YEAST

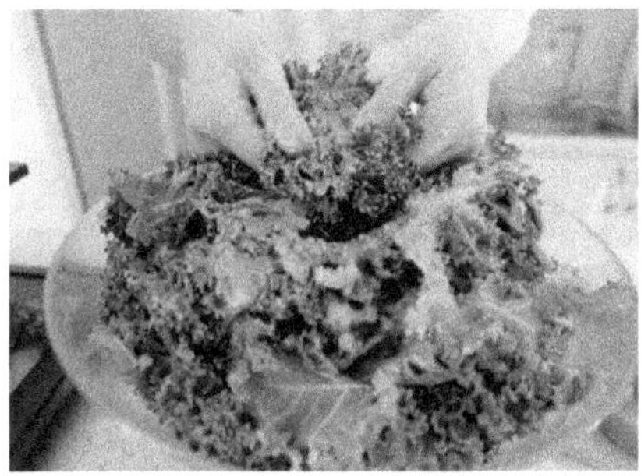

Ingredients for kale chips

Fresh kale leaves, olive oil, nutritional yeast, and salt.

Preparation of kale chip with nutritional yeast

The oven should be heated to 275°F (135°C).

Make sure the kale leaves are completely dry after giving them

a good wash.

Remove the kale's stiff stems and tear the leaves into bite-sized

pieces.

Put the shredded kale in a sizable mixing bowl and drizzle with

little olive oil. Toss the kale to evenly distribute the oil on it.

Sprinkle salt and nutritional yeast over the kale chips. Adjust

the amount to your preference (nutritional yeast provides a

cheesy flavor).

The kale chips should be spread out in a single layer on a

baking sheet lined with parchment paper.

Bake the kale chips in the preheated oven for 20 to 25 minutes,

or until they are crispy and beginning to brown.

Remove from the oven, let the kale chips cool for a few

minutes, and then savor your own homemade chips.

MIXED NUTS AND DRIED FRUITS TRAIL MIX

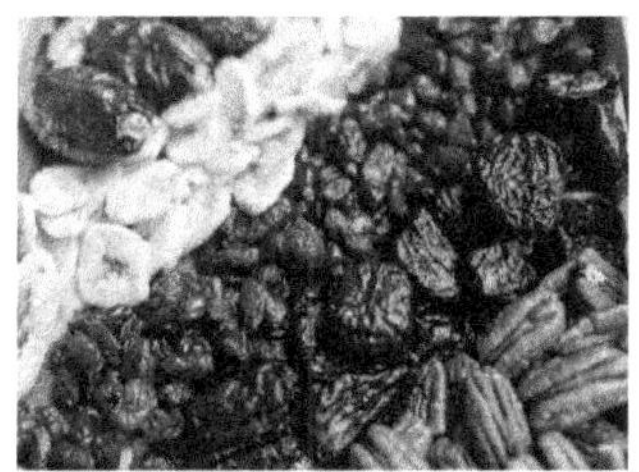

Ingredients for mixed nut and dried fruit

Mixed nuts (almonds, walnuts, cashews), Dried fruits (raisins, cranberries, apricots), Optional additions (seeds, dark chocolate chips, spices)

Preparation of mixed nut and dried fruit

Take out the desired amount of mixed nuts and dried fruit.

Mix any additional spices or herbs with the nuts and dried fruits if you're adding them.

Toss the ingredients together in a big bowl after combining them all.

Place the trail mix in an airtight container to make it simple to enjoy a convenient and healthy snack whenever you want.

VEGETABLE CRUDITÉ PLATTER WITH HUMMUS

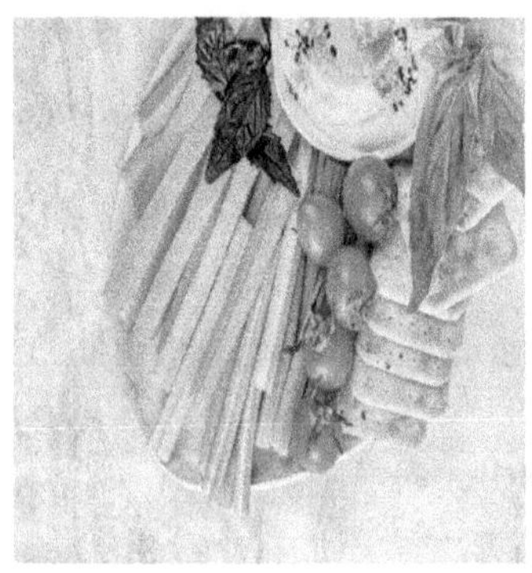

Ingredients

Assorted fresh vegetables (carrot sticks, cucumber slices, bell pepper strips, cherry tomatoes, celery) etc.

Hummus (store-bought or home made)

Procedure

Fresh vegetables should be washed and sliced into bite-sized sticks, slices, or pieces.

Place the vegetarian items in a serving dish or platter.

Provide a dish of hummus in the center for dipping along with the vegetable crudité platter.

Dip the vegetables in the hummus to enjoy this crunchy and healthy snack.

BAKED POTATO FRIES

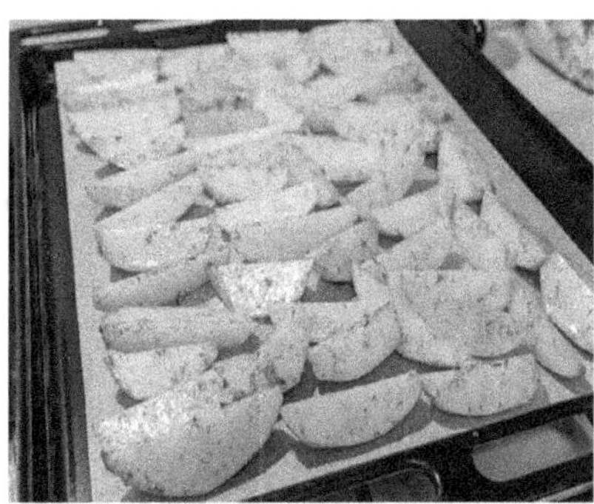

Ingredients

Sweet potatoes, Olive oil, Salt and pepper, Optional spices (paprika, garlic powder).

Procedure

The oven should be heated to 425°F (220°C).

Cut the sweet potatoes into thin strips or wedges after peeling them.

Sweet potato strips should be mixed with olive oil, pepper, salt

and any additional seasonings you choose in a bowl.

The sweet potato fries should be spread out in a single layer on

a baking sheet lined with parchment paper.

Bake the fries in the preheated oven for 20 to 30 minutes,

flipping them over halfway through, or until they are golden brown and crispy.

Take them out of the oven, allow them to cool somewhat, and then enjoy your own homemade baked sweet potato fries.

QUINOA SALAD

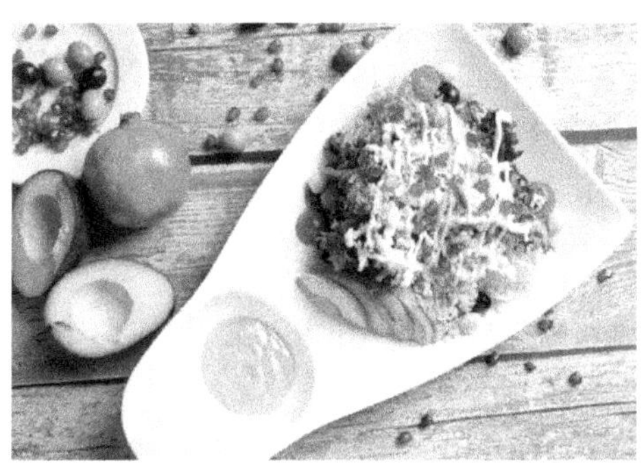

Ingredients

Cooked quinoa, assorted finely chopped vegetables (cucumber,

bell peppers, cherry tomatoes), Fresh herbs (cilantro, parsley),

Dressing (olive oil, lemon juice, salt, pepper), (olives, avocado)

Optional additions

Procedure

Quinoa should be prepared as directed on the package, and then allowed to cool.

Combine cooked and cooled quinoa with finely chopped vegetables and fresh herbs in a bowl.

Prepare dressing by combining olive oil,

 lemon juice, salt, and pepper. It should be drizzled over the quinoa salad and combined.

Add ingredients like olives or avocado for more flavor and creaminess, if desired.

Serve the quinoa salad in miniature cups or bowls as a tasty and healthy snack.

VEGAN SPINACH AND ARTICHOKE DIP

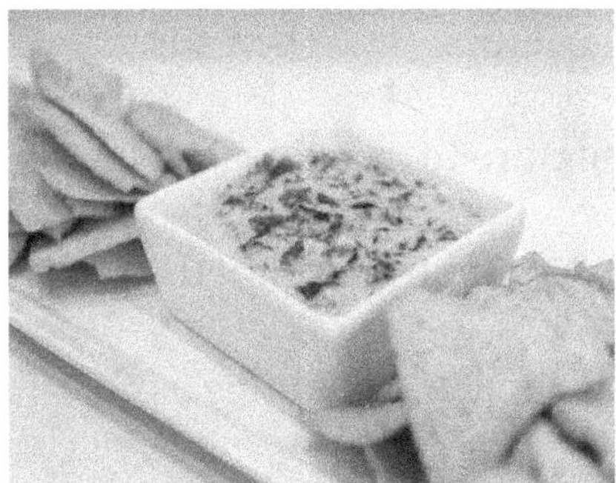

Ingredient for Vegan Spinach and Artichoke dip

1 cup frozen spinach, thawed and drained, 1 cup canned

Artichoke hearts, chopped, 1 cup vegan cream cheese, ½

cup, Vegan mayonnaise, 1/2 cup vegan shredded cheese

(optional), 1/4 cup nutritional yeast (for a cheesy flavor), 2

cloves garlic, Minced, Salt and pepper to taste.

Procedure

The thawed and drained spinach, chopped artichoke hearts,

Vegan cream cheese, vegan mayonnaise, vegan crumbled

Cheese, nutritional yeast, minced garlic, salt, and pepper

should all be combined in a mixing dish.

To thoroughly combine, and then stir.

Transfer the mixture to a baking dish that is oven-safe.

Bake for 25 to 30 minutes or until the top is gently browned

and the dip is heated and bubbling, at 350°F (175°C).

Serving suggestions for the vegan spinach and artichoke dip

include tortilla chips, vegetable sticks, or crusty bread.

STUFFED BELL PEPPERS WITH RICE AND VEGGIES

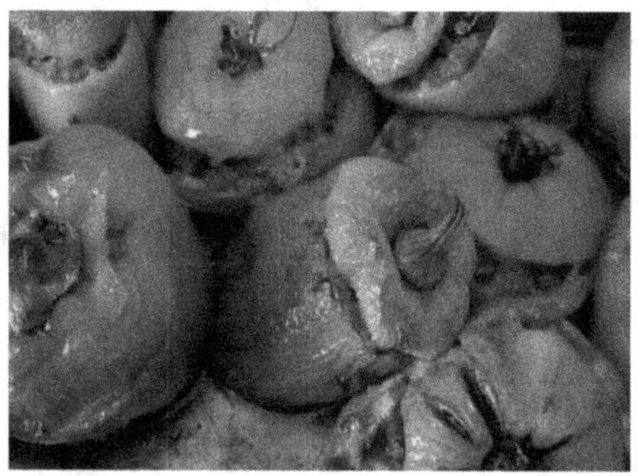

Ingredients

Assorted Bell peppers, Cooked rice (white or brown),

finely chopped vegetables (onion, carrot, zucchini, corn),

Tomato sauce or marinara sauce, Spices and seasonings (garlic

powder, paprika, oregano, salt, and pepper).

Procedure

Cut the bell pepper tops off, then remove the seeds and

membranes.

Finely chopped vegetables should be sautéed in a skillet with

a little olive oil until tender.

Your choice of spices and seasonings should be added to the

skillet along with cooked rice and tomato sauce. Mix well.

Fill each bell pepper with the tasty vegetable mixture.

The stuffed bell peppers should be placed in a baking dish.

To prevent sticking, add a little water to the bottom of the

dish

and cover with foil.

Bake at 350°F (175°C) in a preheated oven for 30-35 minutes,

 or until the bell peppers are tender.

Serve the stuffed bell peppers hot, if desired, with fresh herbs on top.

VEGAN SPRING ROLLS WITH PEANUT DIPPING SAUCE

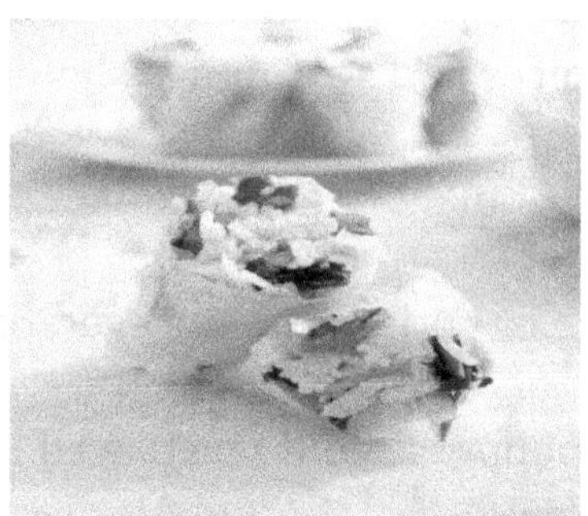

Ingredients for Spring Rolls

Rice paper wrappers, thin rice noodles, cooked and cooled,

Fresh herbs (e. g., mint, cilantro), Assorted vegetables (lettuce, cucumber, bell pepper, carrot), Tofu or tempeh (optional,

marinated and cooked), Avocado slices (optional)

Ingredients for Peanut Dipping Sauce

Peanut butter, Soy sauce or tamari, Lime juice, Maple syrup or

Agave nectar, Water, Crushed red pepper flakes (optional).

Procedure for Spring Rolls

A rice paper wrapper should be softened by being dipped in

Warm water before being placed on a clean, wet kitchen

towel.

In the center of the wrapper, place a small amount of cooked

rice noodles, fresh herbs, slices of vegetables, and any

additional ingredients you want to use, such as tofu or

avocado.

Like a burrito, roll the wrapper tightly after folding the sides

over the filling.   continue by adding the remaining

ingredients.

Procedure for Peanut Dipping Sauce

To achieve the desired consistency, combine the following

 ingredients in a bowl: pecan butter, soy sauce or tamari, lime

Juice, maple syrup or agave nectar, and a little water.

Crushed red pepper flakes can be used for some heat.

For a refreshing and tasty snack, serve the vegan spring rolls

with the peanut dipping sauce.

VEGAN SPINACH AND MUSHROOM STUFFED MUSHROOMS

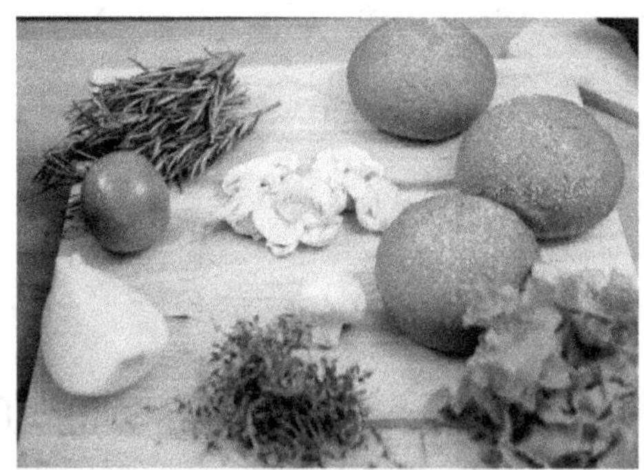

Ingredients

Large mushroom caps (cremini or button mushrooms), Fresh spinach, chopped, Mushrooms, finely chopped, Onion, finely chopped, Garlic, minced, Vegan bread crumbs, Vegan cream cheese or vegan sour cream, Nutritional yeast (for a cheesy flavor), Spices and herbs (thyme, oregano, salt, and pepper).

Procedure

Take the stems out of the mushroom caps and place them side by side.

Chopped mushroom stems, onion, and garlic should be sautéed

 in a skillet until tender.

Chop up some spinach and add it after.

Remove too much moisture.

Add nutritional yeast, bread crumbs, vegan cream cheese or

 vegan sour cream, as well as your preferred spices and herbs.

Put the spinach and mushroom mixture inside the mushroom caps.

The stuffed mushrooms should be placed on a baking sheet.

Cook for 20 to 25 minutes, or until the mushrooms are tender

 and the tops are gently browned, in a preheated oven at 375°F (190°C).

Serve the vegan stuffed mushrooms as an appetizer or snack.

VEGAN BUFFALO CAULIFLOWER BITES

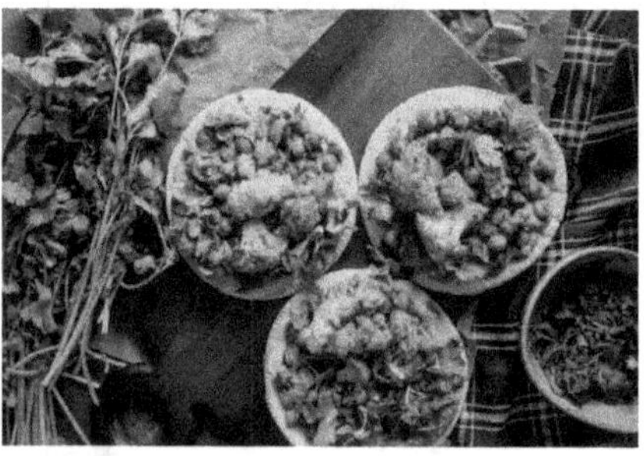

Ingredients

Cauliflower florets, Gluten-free Flour, Water or plant-based milk, Buffalo sauce, Vegan butter or margarine, Spices (garlic powder, onion powder, paprika, salt, and pepper).

Procedure

To make a thick batter, mix gluten free flour with water or plant-based milk in a bowl.

Make sure the cauliflower flowers are thoroughly coated by

dipping them into the batter.

Place the coated cauliflower on a baking sheet with parchment

paper between the layers.

Cook the cauliflower for 20 to 25 minutes at 450°F (230°C), or until it is crisp and lightly browned.

Procedure of buffalo sauce

Melt vegan butter or margarine in a pot.

Taste the buffalo sauce and seasonings (salt, pepper, paprika, onion powder, garlic powder).

Simmer for a few minutes while stirring to thoroughly combine and heat the sauce.

Make sure the baked cauliflower is evenly coated before tossing it in the buffalo sauce.

Provide vegan ranch or blue cheese dressing for dipping along

with the vegan buffalo cauliflower bites.

VEGAN CHOCOLATE AVOCADO MOUSSE

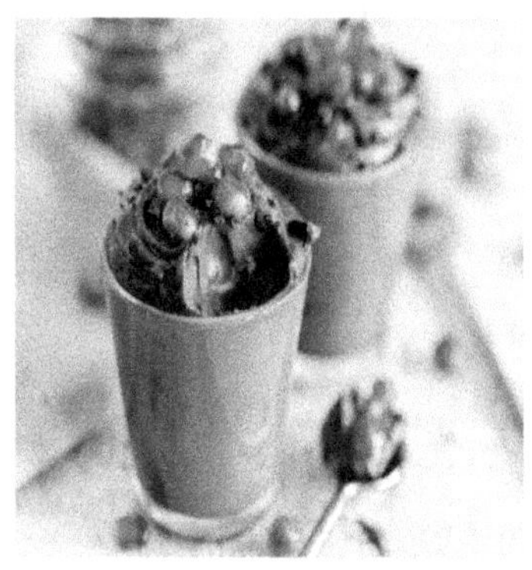

Ingredients

2 Ripe avocados, Cocoa powder, Maple syrup or agave nectar

Vanilla extract, a pinch of salt, berries or chopped nuts (Optional toppings).

Procedure

Scoop the ripe avocados' flesh into a food processor or blender.

To the blender, add cocoa powder, maple syrup or agave nectar, vanilla extract, and a dash of salt.

Blend the mixture until it is creamy and smooth, scraping the sides as necessary.

Taste and add more maple syrup or cocoa powder to achieve the desired sweetness or chocolate flavor.

Transfer the chocolate avocado mousse to serving dishes, and top with your preferred garnish, such as chopped almonds or berries.

Refrigerate for a few hours or serve right away for a decadent chocolate dessert.

ENERGY BITES WITH DATES AND NUTS

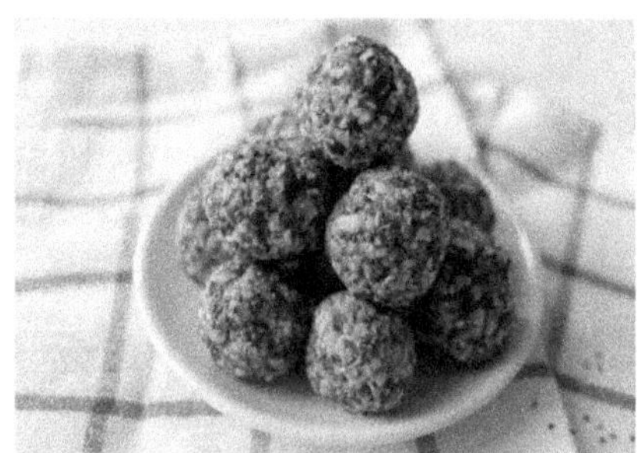

Ingredients

Dates, pitted, Nuts (almonds, cashews, or a mix), Rolled oats,

Chia seeds or flaxseeds., Coconut flakes, Nut butter (almond or

peanut butter), Vanilla extract, Cocoa powder, cinnamon,

dried fruits (Optional add-ins).

Procedure

In a food processor, combine the dates and nuts until they

create a crumbly, sticky mixture.

Rolling oats, chia or flax seeds, coconut flakes, nut butter, vanilla extract, and any additional ingredients are added to the

food processor.

Repeat the process until everything is thoroughly mixed and

the mixture holds together when called for.

Roll the little bits into bite-sized balls by scooping them out.

The energy bites should be chilled for at least 30 minutes to

firm up.

Enjoy these wholesome and portable sweet treats once they

have chilled.

VEGAN BERRY PARFAIT

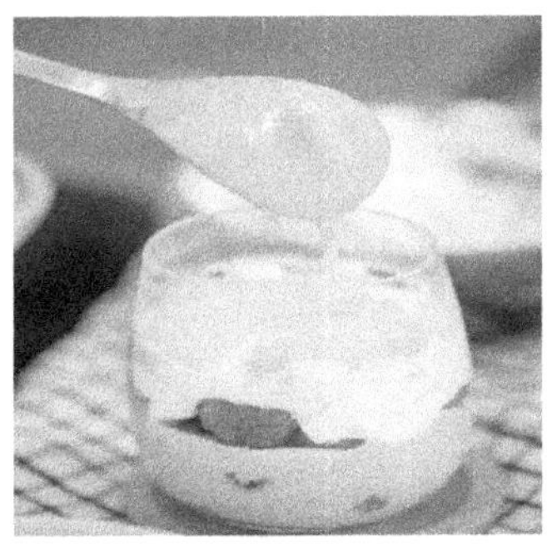

Ingredients

Vegan yogurt (almond, soy, or coconut), Fresh berries (strawberries, blueberries, raspberries), Granola, Maple syrup

or agave nectar (Optional sweetener).

Procedure

In a glass or bowl, layer vegan yogurt with fresh berries.

Add a layer of granola for crunch and texture.

Drizzle a small amount of optional sweetener (maple syrup or agave nectar) if desired.

Repeat the layers until you've created your parfait.

Top with a few more berries for a vibrant and delightful vegan berry parfait.

BANANA ICE CREAM WITH VARIOUS TOPPINGS

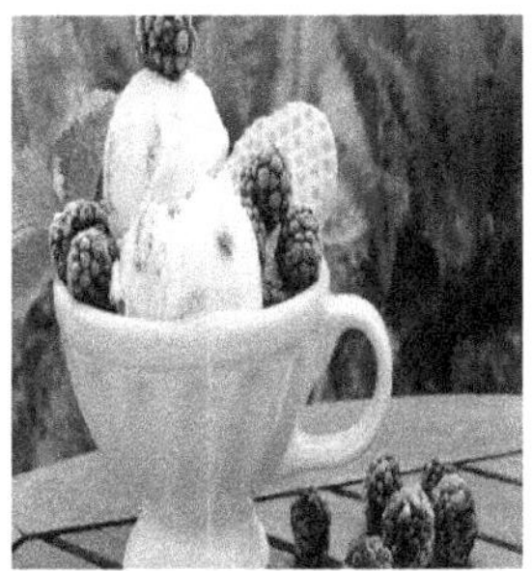

Ingredients

Ripe bananas, sliced and frozen, Optional toppings (chopped

nuts, chocolate chips, coconut flakes, berries)

Procedure

Place the frozen banana slices in a food processor.

Blend the bananas until they turn creamy and smooth,

resembling ice cream.

You may need to stop and scrape down the sides as you go.

Once the banana ice cream is smooth, transfer it to a bowl.

Add your choice of toppings such as chopped nuts, chocolate

chips, coconut flakes, or berries etc.

Refrigerate Serve the banana ice-cream immediately as a

simple and healthy dessert.

VEGAN OATMEAL COOKIES

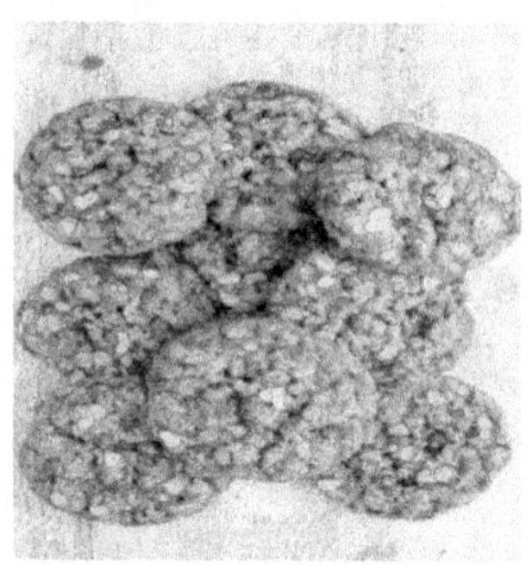

Ingredients

Rolled oats, Gluten-free Flour baking soda, Vegan butter or

 coconut oil, Brown sugar or coconut sugar, Flaxseed meal (egg

substitute), Vanilla extract, Optional add-ins (raisins, chocolate

chips, nuts).

Procedure

Rolling oats, flour, and baking soda should all be combined in a mixing basin.

Blend vegan butter or coconut oil with brown sugar or coconut sugar in a separate bowl.

Add vanilla extract and flaxseed meal mixed with water (egg substitute) to the dry ingredients, blend until uniform.

As you gradually incorporate the dry ingredients into the wet ingredients, mix until a doughy consistency develops.

Add any extras, like as raisins, chocolate chips, or nuts, by folding them in.

Cookie dough should be spooned out onto a baking sheet that has been lined with parchment paper.

Cookies should be baked for 10 to 12 minutes at 350°F (175°C) or until golden brown.

Before enjoying these delicious vegan oatmeal cookies, let them cool on a wire rack.

ZUCCHINI CHIPS WITH A DILL DIP

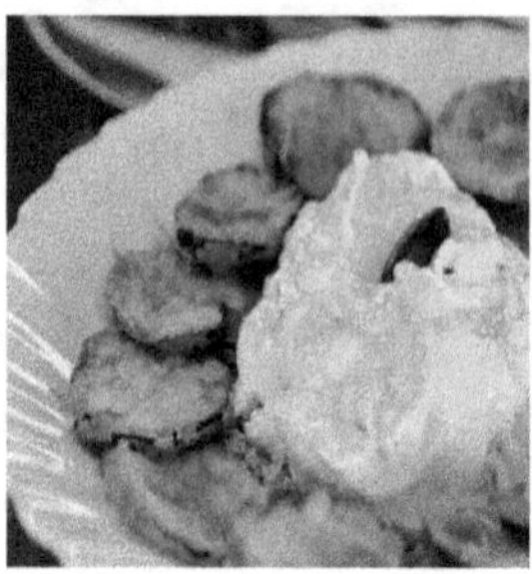

Ingredients

Zucchini, thinly sliced, Gluten-free bread crumbs or almond meal, Olive oil or cooking spray, Salt and pepper, Fresh dill (for the dip), Vegan yogurt or vegan sour cream (for the dip), Lemon juice (for the dip), garlic powder (for the dip).

Procedure for Zucchini Chips

The oven should be heated to 425°F (220°C).

Sliced zucchini should be briefly tossed in olive oil or sprayed with cooking spray after being thinly sliced.

Sprinkle salt and pepper on the zucchini slices before coating them with gluten-free bread crumbs or almond meal.

Place the coated zucchini slices in a single layer on a baking sheet.

Bake the zucchini chips for 20 to 25 minutes, or until they are crispy and golden brown.

Procedure for Dill Dip

Put vegan yogurt or vegan sour cream, chopped fresh dill, lemon juice, and a pinch of garlic powder in a bowl.

To thoroughly combine, stir.

Serving the zucchini chips with the dill dip will result in a tasty vegan snack that is gluten-free.

CHICKPEA FLOUR PANCAKES WITH VEGAN CHEESE

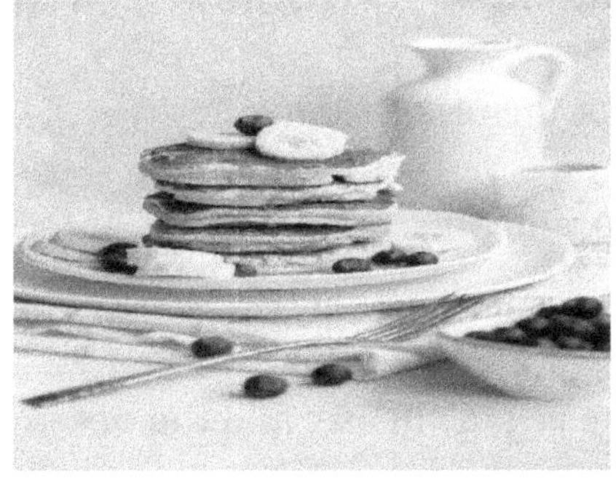

Ingredients

Chickpea flour, Water, Salt and pepper, Vegan cheese shreds or

slices, Vegetable oil, Toppings (optional).

Procedure

To make a thick cake batter, combine chickpea flour, water,

salt, and pepper in a bowl.

A non-stick skillet or frying pan should be heated over

Medium-high heat with some cooking oil added.

A ladleful of the chickpea flour batter should be poured onto

 the hot skillet to create a pancake.

sear the bottom till golden brown and crisp before flipping it

over to sear the other side.

Once both sides of the pancake are cooked, top one with

vegan cheese slices or shreds.

To melt the vegan cheese, fold the bread in half.

Remove the cake from the heat and slice it into wedges or

triangles.

Serve these vegan chickpea flour pancakes with melted cheese and a drizzle of sauce as a delicious snack.

GLUTEN-FREE VEGAN BROWNIES

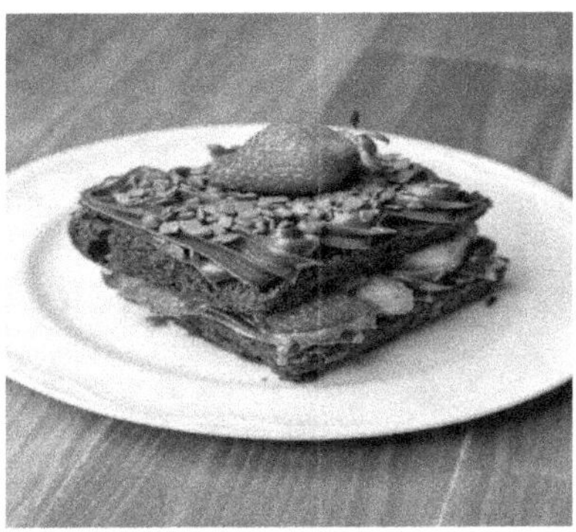

Ingredients

Gluten free all purpose flour or almond flour, Cocoa powder,

Baking powder, Salt, Vegan butter or coconut oil, Sugar

coconut, Flaxseed meal mixed with water (egg substitute),

Vanilla extract, Vegan chocolate chips (gluten-free

Procedure

Combine gluten-free flour, baking powder, cocoa powder, and

salt in a mixing bowl.

Cream sugar and vegan butter or coconut oil in a separate bowl.

Add vanilla extract and flaxseed meal mixed with water

 (Egg substitute) to the dry ingredients, blend until uniform.

The dry ingredients should be added gradually to the wet

ingredients, then combined thoroughly by stirring.

include the vegan chocolate chips.

Transfer the battery to a baking pan with a grated and lined surface.

Bake for 20 to 25 minutes at 350 °F (175 °C) or until a

Tooth-pick inserted into the center comes out with a few wet crumbs.

Before cutting the brownies into squares allow them to cool.

 Enjoy these vegan brownies without gluten as a sweet treat!

VEGAN NACHOS WITH HOMEMADE CASHEW CHEESE

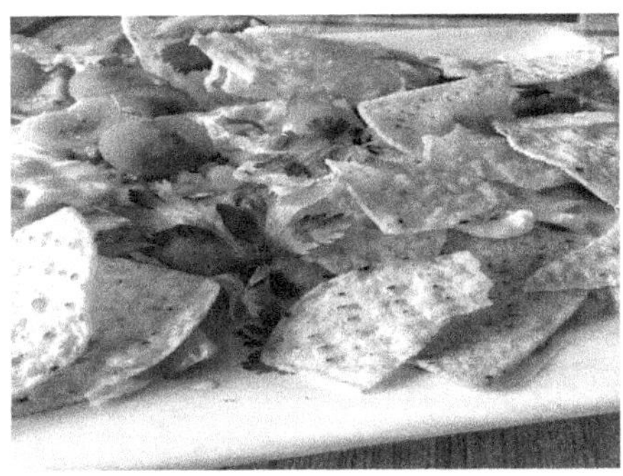

Ingredients for Cashew Cheese Sauce

1 cup raw cashews, soaked and drained, 1/4 cup nutritional

yeast, 1/4 cup water, 2 tablespoons lemon juice, 1 clove garlic

1/2 teaspoon salt.

Ingredients for Nachos

Vegan Tortilla chips, Black beans, cooked and seasoned,

Sliced jalapeños (optional), Chopped tomatoes, Sliced black

olives, Chopped green onions, Guacamole (optional), Salsa.

Procedure for Cashew Cheese Sauce

Cashews that have been soaked and drained, nutritional yeast,

water, lemon juice, garlic, and salt should all be put in a blender.

If additional water is required to get the desired consistency, blend until the product is smooth and creamy.

Procedures for Nachos

Arrange tortilla chips on a serving platter.

Drizzle the homemade cashew cheese sauce over the chips.

Add seasoned black beans, jalapeños (if desired), chopped tomatoes, sliced black olives, and chopped green onions.

Optionally, serve with guacamole and salsa on the side.

Serve the vegan nachos as a delicious and indulgent party snack

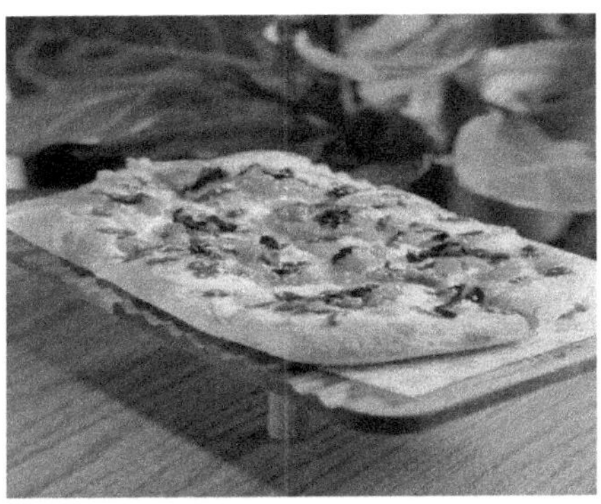

Ingredients for Pizza Dough

Gluten-free all purpose flour, Yeast, Warm water, Olive oil, Salt and Sugar.

For Toppings

Vegan pizza sauce, Vegan cheese shreds, Sliced vegetables (bell

peppers, cherry tomatoes, and olives), Vegan pepperoni slices

(optional)

Procedure for Pizza Dough

If making homemade dough, mix flour, yeast, warm water,

olive oil, salt, and a pinch of sugar to activate the yeast.

Knead the dough until its smooth and elastic, and then let it rise until doubled in size.

Procedure for Mini Pizza Bites

Set your oven to the temperature that your pizza dough requires.

Pizza dough should be rolled out and cut into little rounds with a glass or cookie cutter.

Pizza sauce, vegan cheese crumbles, cut vegetables, and vegan pepperoni (if preferred) should be sprinkled on top of each round.

Bake in the preheated oven until the cheese is bubbling and the dough is golden brown.

For your special occasion, serve the vegan small pizza slices as bite-sized snacks.

CONCLUSION

In addition to being a collection of recipes, "25 Healthy Vegan Snacks Cookbook" is a celebration of the imagination, kindness, and dedication of those who chose a vegan lifestyle. By taking this culinary tour, we have experienced new tastes and provided our bodies with healthy, plant-based nutrients.

You've found a wide variety of snack ideas in these pages, from spicy to sweet, simple to decadent. The beauty of veganism is reflected in these dishes, which are not seen as a sacrifice but rather as a celebration of the bounty that nature gives.

We help our own health and the health of the earth when we adopt a vegan diet. We are more conscious of our environmental impact, we use fewer resources, and we respect the lives of animals. The recipes in "25 Healthy Vegan Snacks Cookbook" are proof that going vegan doesn't have to mean giving up on good food.

Please don't stop trying new things, being creative, and discovering exciting new vegan snacks. I hope this cookbook encourages you to make conscious decisions that are good for your health, the animals, and the environment, whether you're a seasoned vegan or just starting out on this path.

Thank you for coming along on this tasty journey with me, and may you find endless happiness in the process of preparing and devouring these wholesome vegan treats.